In celebration of Maeve!
Love Gran

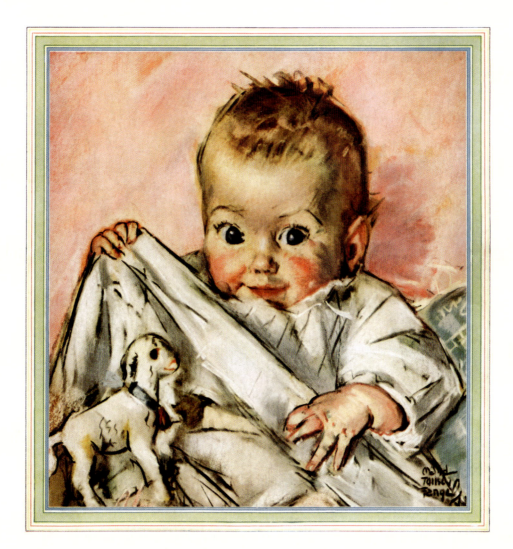

VOTES for BABIES

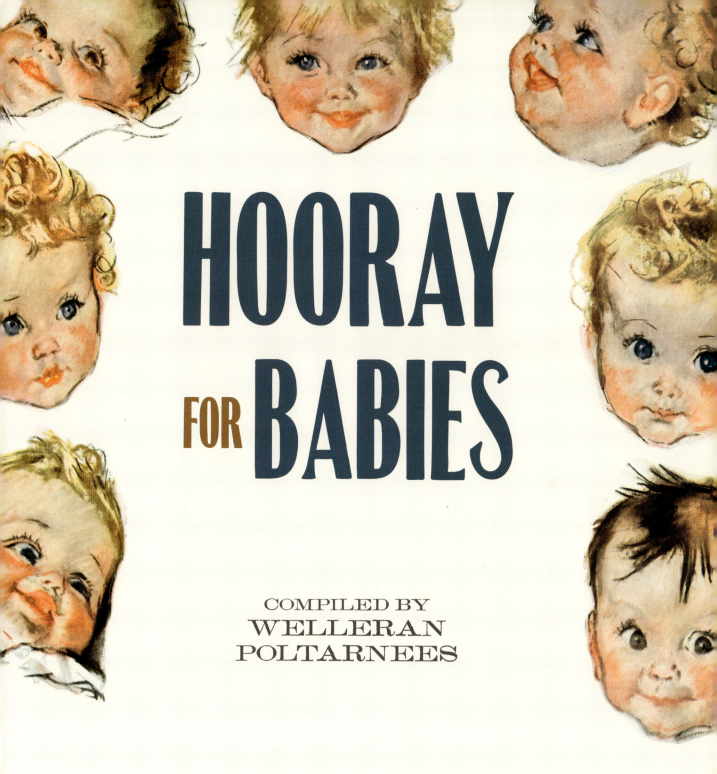

HOORAY FOR BABIES

COMPILED BY
WELLERAN POLTARNEES

LAUGHING ELEPHANT · MMX

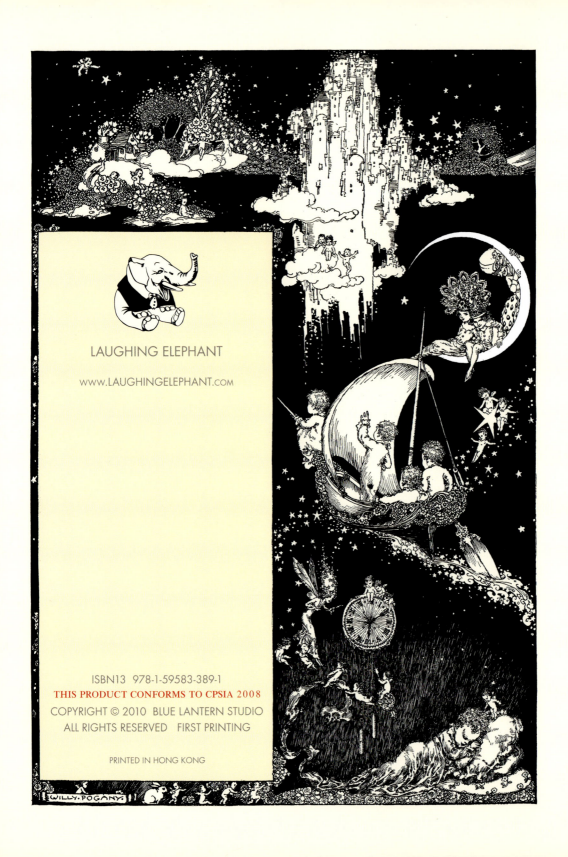

LAUGHING ELEPHANT

www.LAUGHINGELEPHANT.com

ISBN13 978-1-59583-389-1
THIS PRODUCT CONFORMS TO CPSIA 2008
COPYRIGHT © 2010 BLUE LANTERN STUDIO
ALL RIGHTS RESERVED FIRST PRINTING

PRINTED IN HONG KONG

Introduction

Look into a baby's eyes. Look long and openly, what you will see is humanity's basic self. You see innocence, openness, curiosity, vulnerability, and, above all, a need for love. This is how we all were before the events of growing up formed the elaborate disguises that we wear. In contemplating babyhood we refresh ourselves, we remind ourselves of what we were, and which we still have buried within.

Compiling this book has been a delightful task. I have turned the pages of our large collection of baby record books. I have reviewed hundreds of magazine illustrations. I have combed our postcard collection. I have reviewed many hundreds of quotations about babies. All of this has touched me and I hope that my selection of words and images will touch you.

WELLERAN POLTARNEES

The WONDER of Their Being

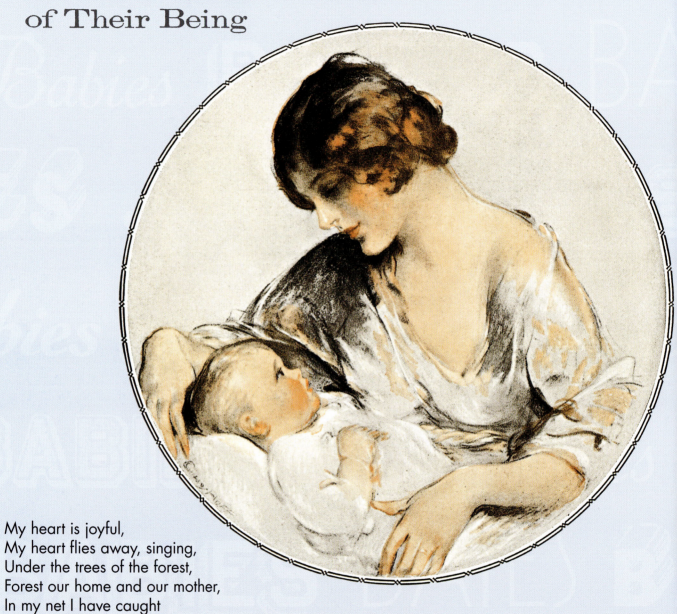

My heart is joyful,
My heart flies away, singing,
Under the trees of the forest,
Forest our home and our mother,
In my net I have caught
A little bird.
My heart is caught in the net,
In the net with the bird.

WESTERN AFRICAN FOLKSONG

WONDER

Frail newborn wings,
Small voice that sings,
New little beating heart,
Dread not thy birth,
Nor fear the earth—
The Infinite thou art:

The sun doth shine,
The earth doth spin.
For welcome— enter in
This green and daisied sphere.
Rejoice— and have no fear.

RICHARD LE GALLIENNE

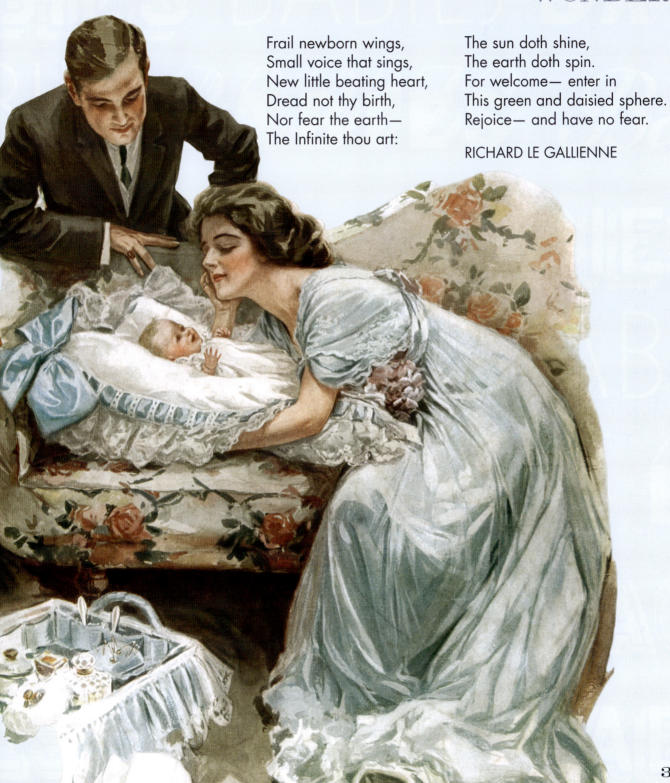

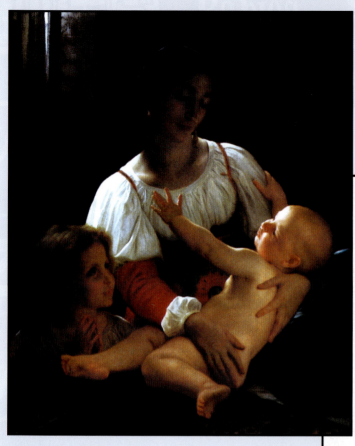
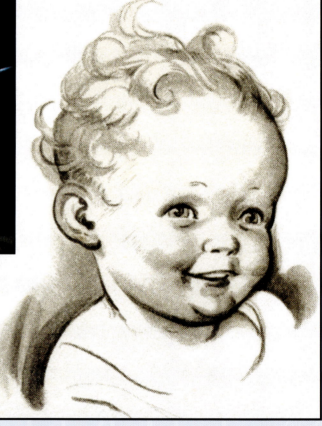

You come from the region of long ago,
    And gazing awhile where the seraphs dwell
Has given your face a glory and glow—
    Of that brighter land have you aught to tell?
I seem to have known it—I more would know,
    Baby mine.

    GEORGE W. CABLE

WONDER

There came to port last Sunday night
  The queerest little craft,
Without an inch of rigging on;
  I looked and looked—and laughed.
It seemed so curious that she
  Should cross the unknown water,
And moor herself within my room—
  My daughter! O, my daughter!

RICHARD LE GALLIENNE

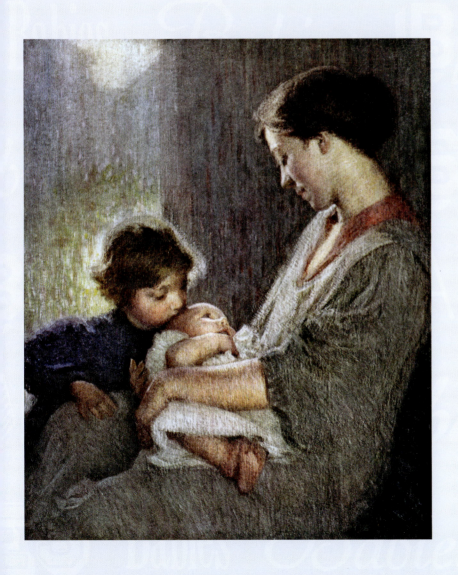

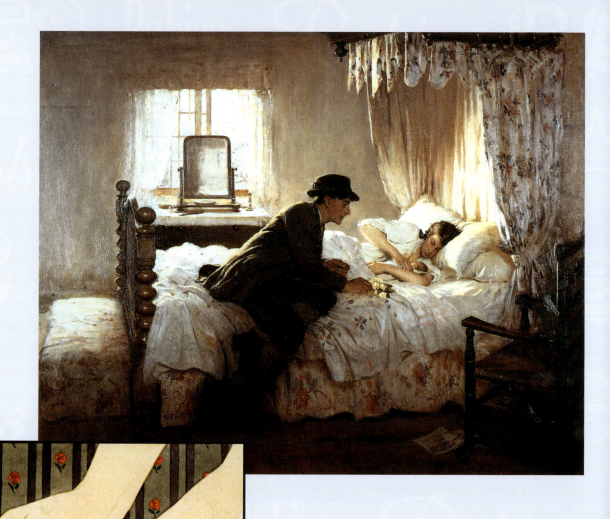

Small traveler from an unseen shore,
By mortal eye ne'er seen before,
To you, good-morrow.

COSMO MONKHOUSE

WONDER

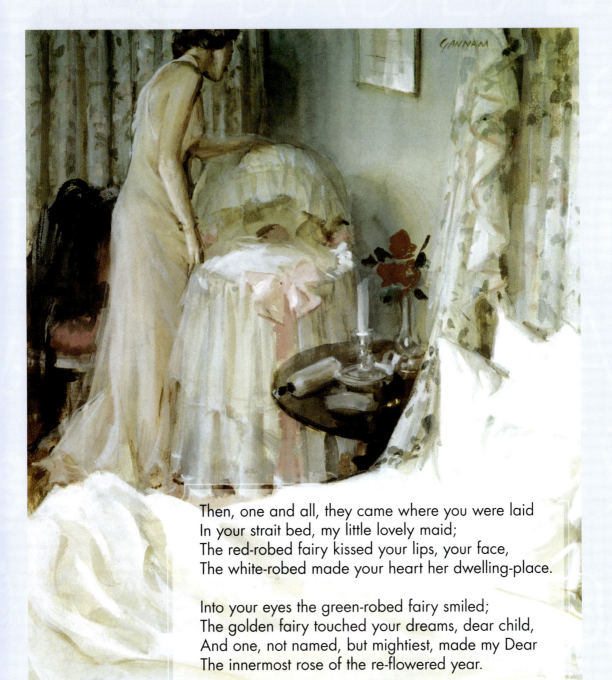

Then, one and all, they came where you were laid
In your strait bed, my little lovely maid;
The red-robed fairy kissed your lips, your face,
The white-robed made your heart her dwelling-place.

Into your eyes the green-robed fairy smiled;
The golden fairy touched your dreams, dear child,
And one, not named, but mightiest, made my Dear
The innermost rose of the re-flowered year.

E. NESBIT

WONDER

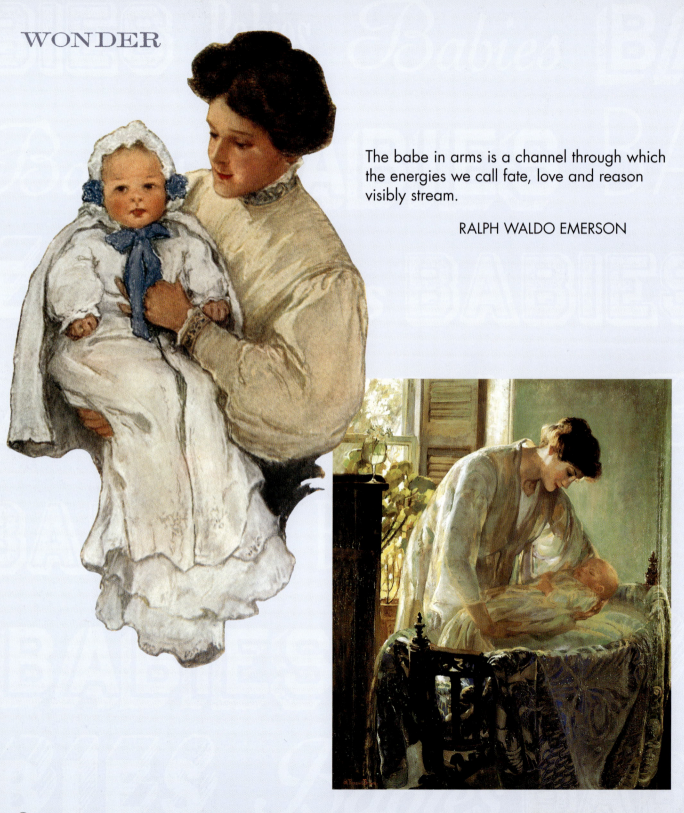

The babe in arms is a channel through which the energies we call fate, love and reason visibly stream.

RALPH WALDO EMERSON

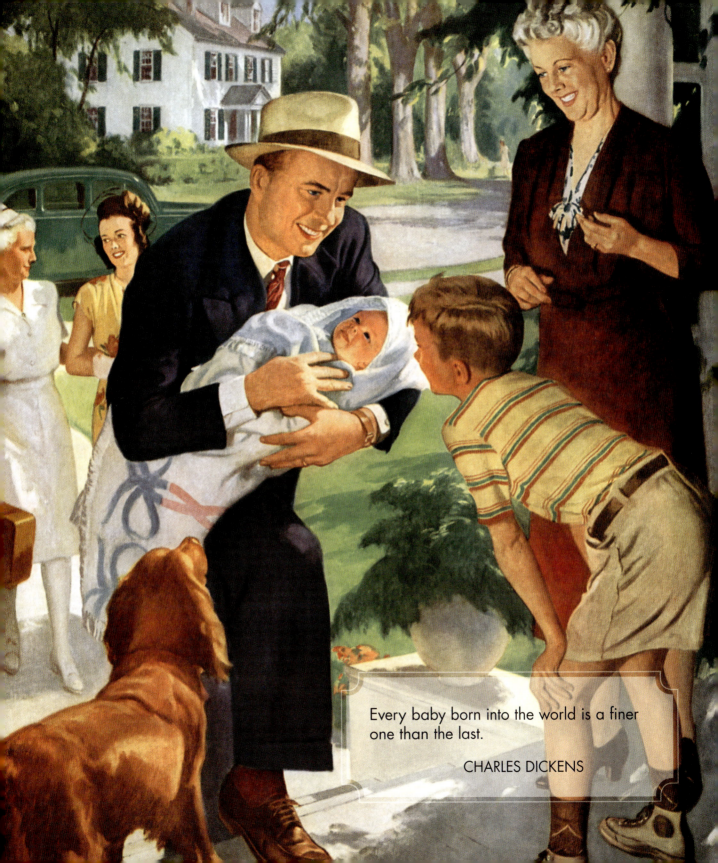

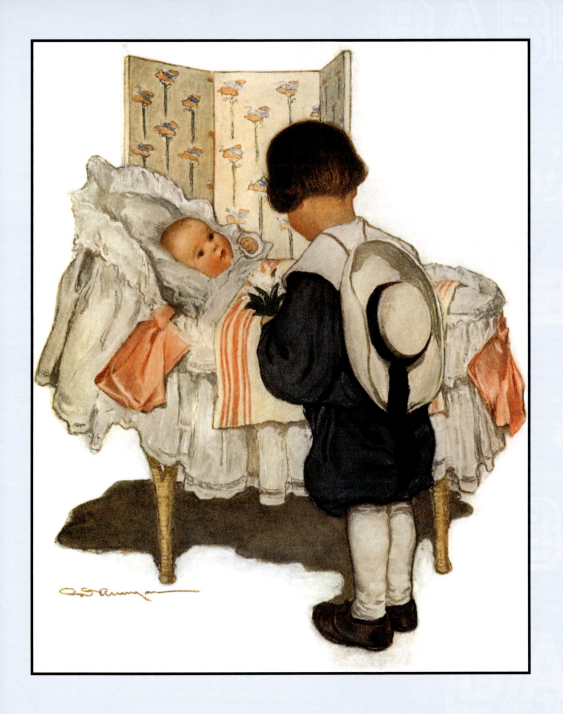

For of all the beings that have ever been since the beginning, Baby is alone the only invincible one.

PENOBSCOT LEGEND

WONDER

Thou straggler into loving arms,
Young climber-up of knees,
When I forget thy thousand ways,
Then life and all shall cease.

MARY ANNE LAMB

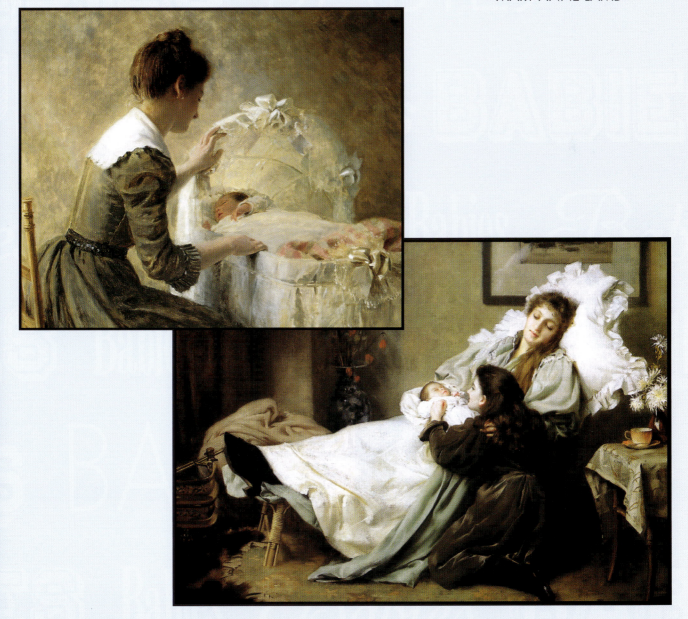

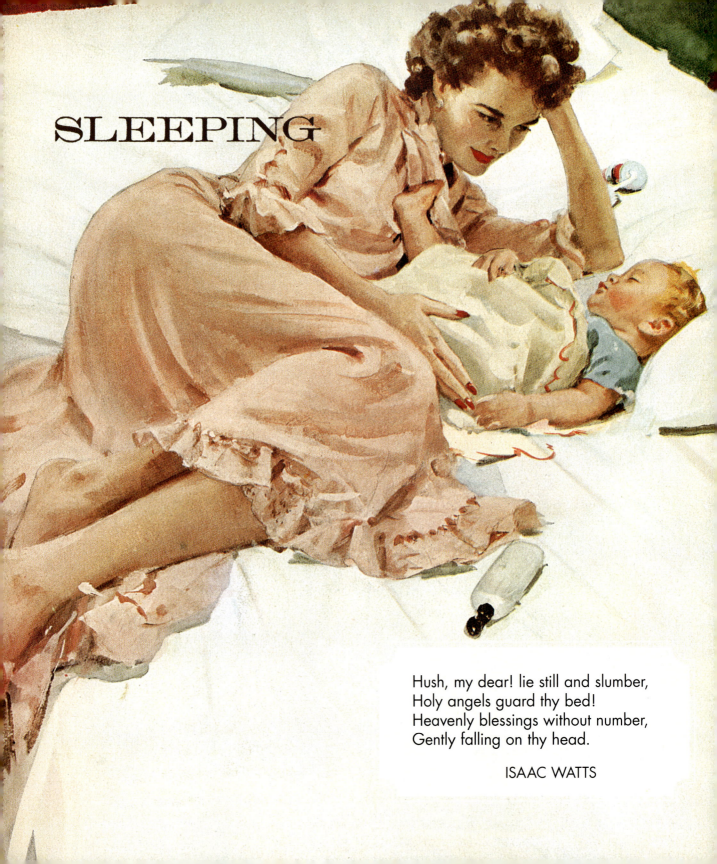

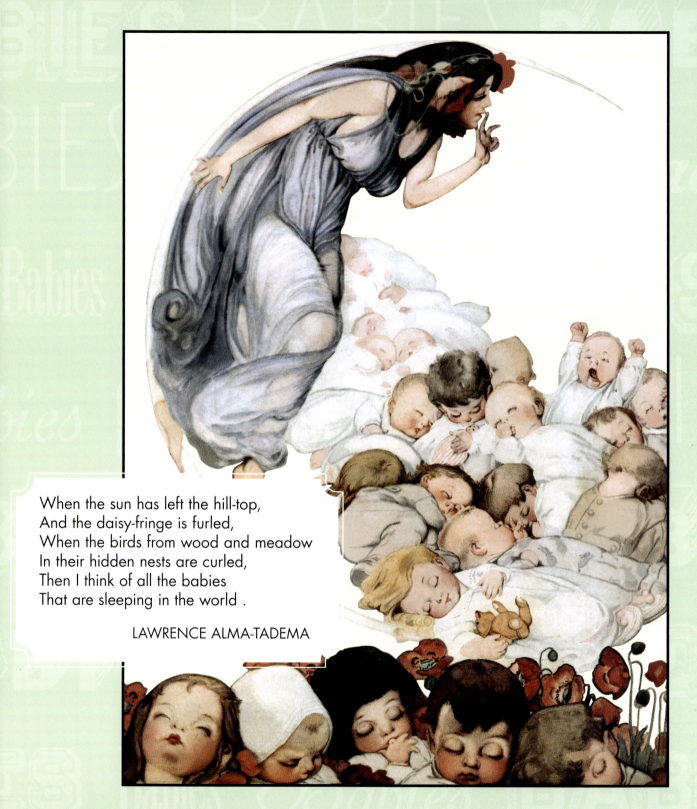

When the sun has left the hill-top,
And the daisy-fringe is furled,
When the birds from wood and meadow
In their hidden nests are curled,
Then I think of all the babies
That are sleeping in the world .

LAWRENCE ALMA-TADEMA

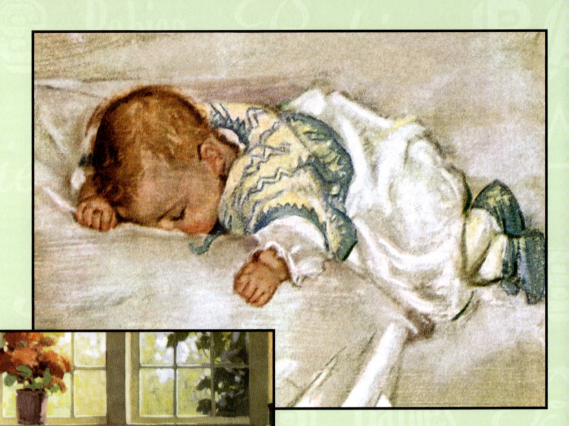

There never was a child so lovely but his mother was glad to get him asleep.

RALPH WALDO EMERSON

SLEEPING

Where has my dear little baby gone?
Gone off to sleepy-land all alone.
What will my dear little baby do?
Play with the dreams, and laugh at them too.
Over in sleepy-land, over and under,

Dreams chase each other away,
Over in dream-land, sleepy eyes wonder,
To see all the dreams at play.
Sleepy-land, dream-land,
Dream-land, sleepy-land,

Dear little baby has gone.

    IDA WAUGH

There he lay upon his back,
The yearling creature, warm and moist with life
To the bottom of his dimples— and to the ends
Of the lovely tumbled curls about his face;
For since he had been covered over-much
To keep him from the light glare, both his cheeks
Were hot and scarlet as the first live rose
The shepherd's heart-blood ebbed away into
The faster for his love. And love was here
As instant; in the pretty baby mouth,
Shut close as if for dreaming that it sucked,
The little naked feet, drawn up the way
Of nestled birdlings; everything so soft
And tender— to the tiny holdfast hands,
Which, closing on a finger into sleep
Had kept the mould of't.

ELIZABETH BARRETT BROWNING

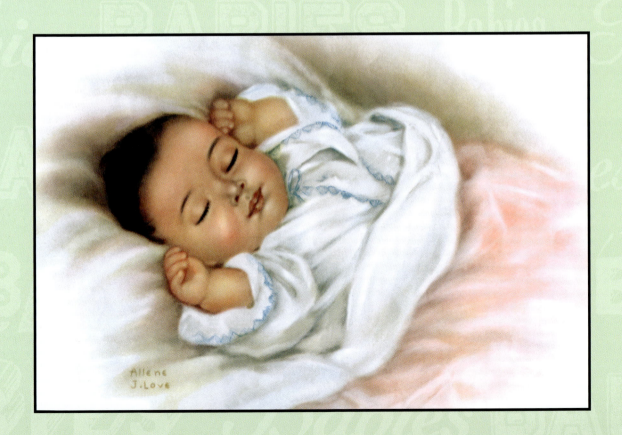

SLEEPING

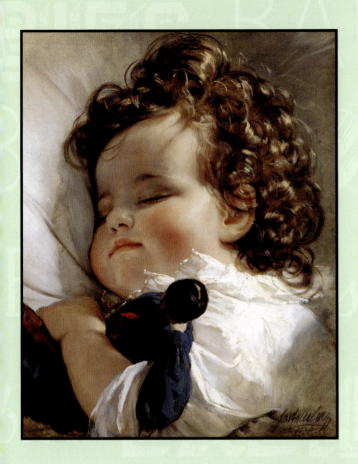

Angels at the foot,
And Angels at the head,
And like a curly little lamb
My pretty babe in bed.

　　　　CHRISTINA ROSSETTI

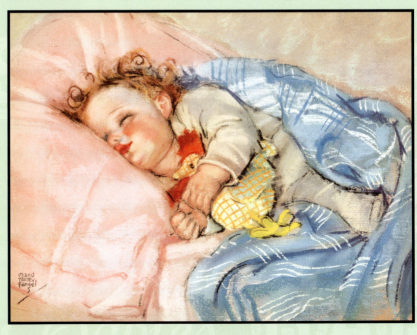

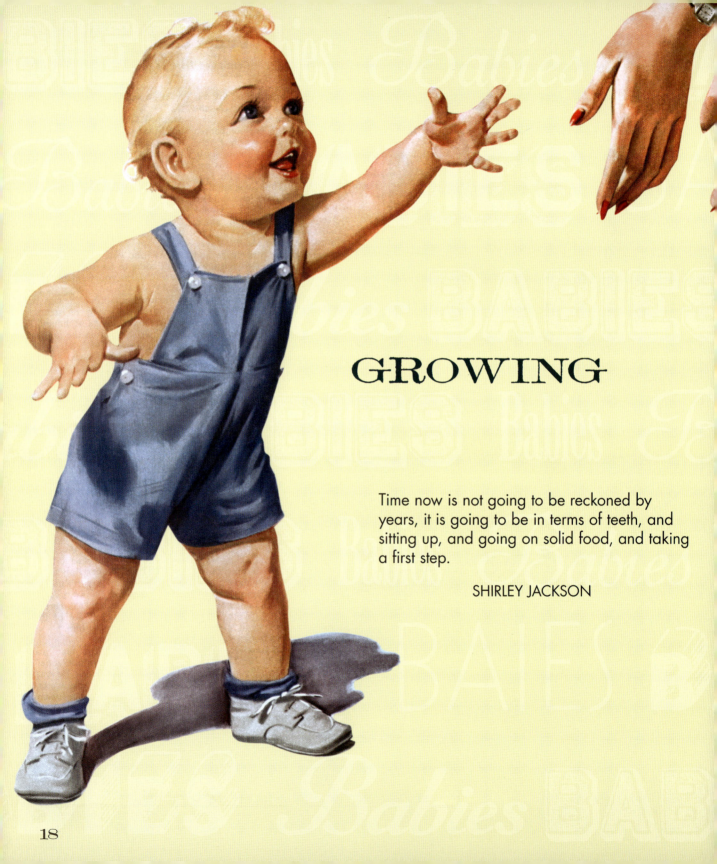

GROWING

Time now is not going to be reckoned by years, it is going to be in terms of teeth, and sitting up, and going on solid food, and taking a first step.

SHIRLEY JACKSON

GROWING

Baby knows all manner of wise words, though
Few on earth can understand their meaning.

It is not for nothing that he never wants to speak.
The one thing he wants to learn is mother's words.

RABINDRANATH TAGORE

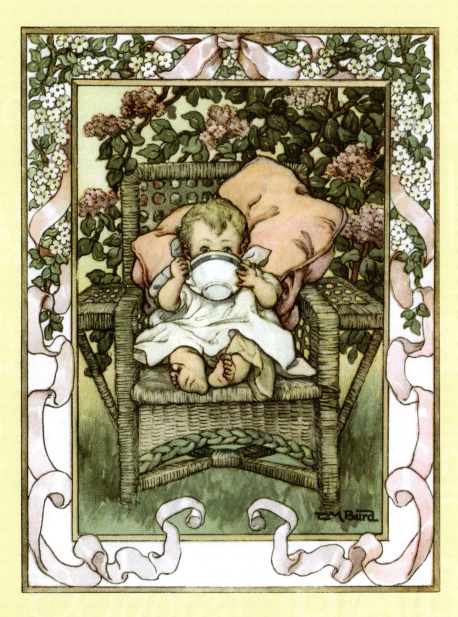

GROWING

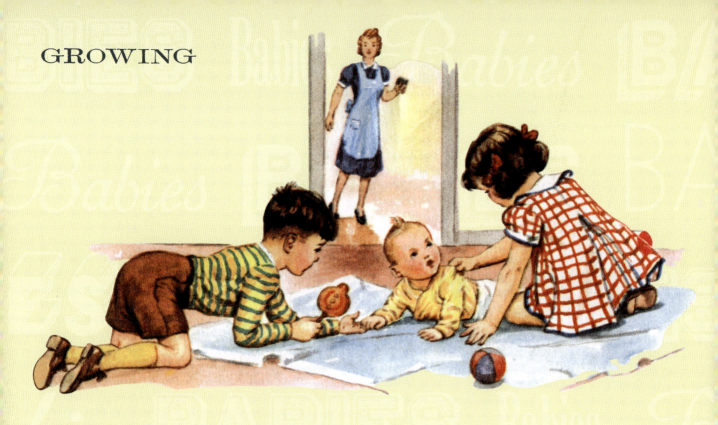

Moving between the legs of tables and of chairs,
Rising or falling, grasping at kisses and toys,
Advancing boldly, sudden to take alarm,
Retreating to the corner of arm and knee,
Eager to be reassured, taking pleasure
In the fragrant brilliance of the Christmas tree.

    T.S. ELIOT

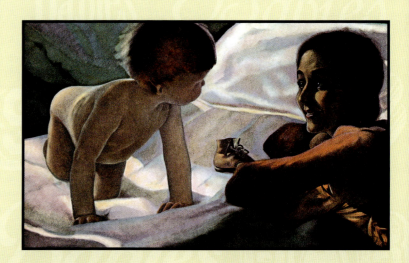

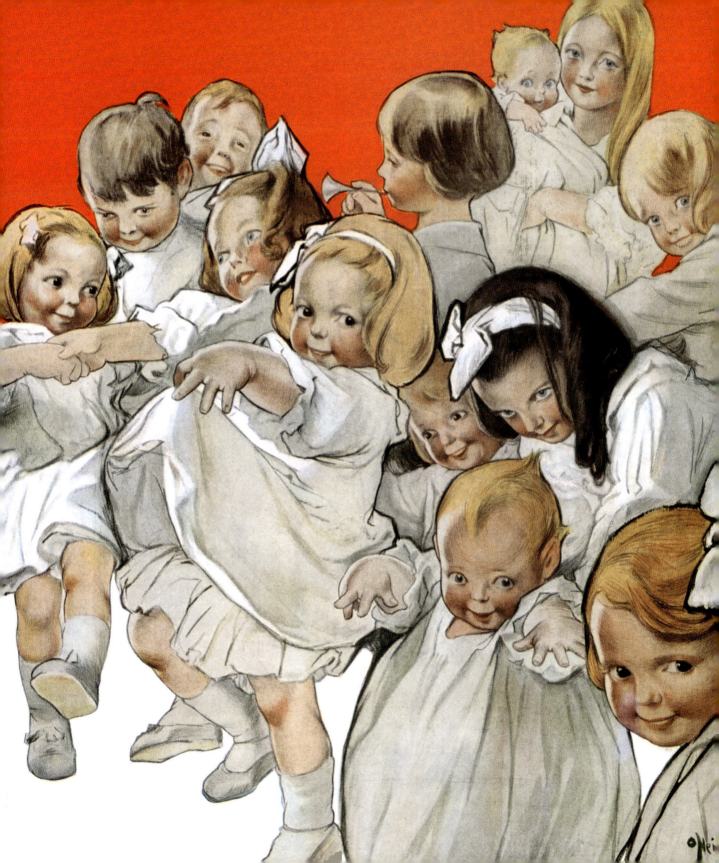

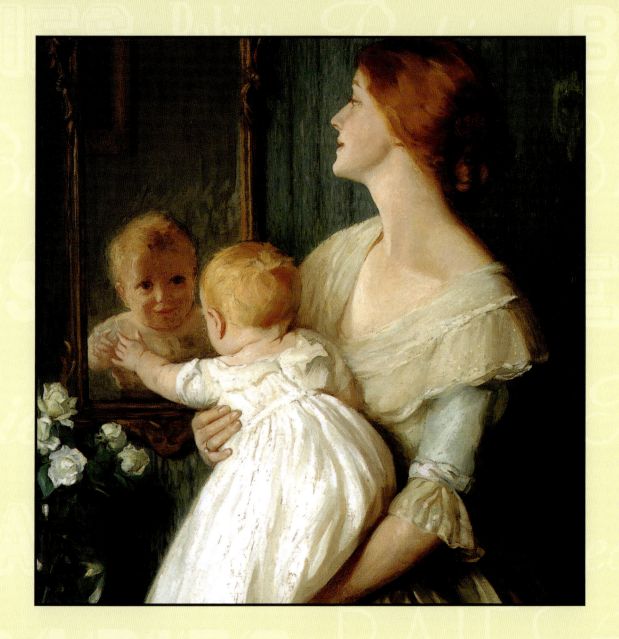

How does the child assimilate his environment? He does it solely in virtue of one of those characteristics that we now know him to have. This is an intense and specialized sensitiveness in consequence of which the things about him awaken so much interest and so much enthusiasm that they become incorporated in his very existence. The child absorbs these impressions not with his mind but with his life itself.

    MARIA MONTESSORI

GROWING

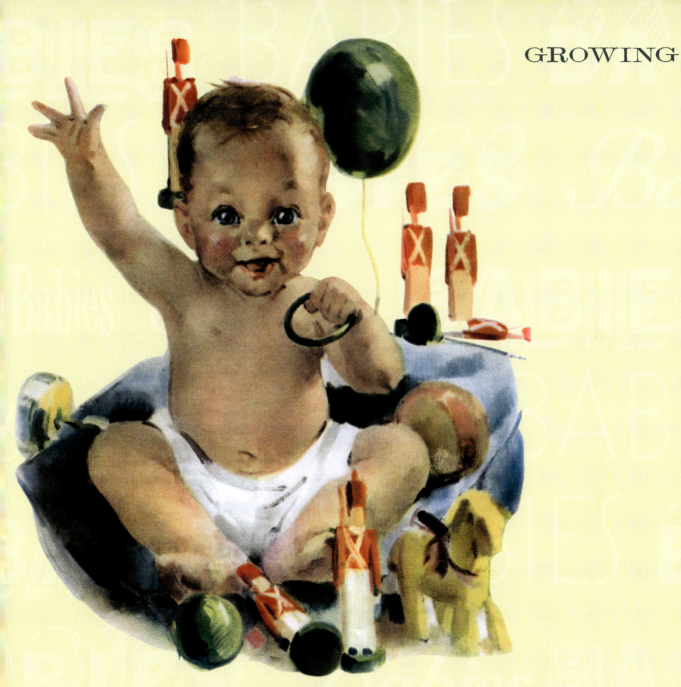

There is something very cheerful and courageous in the setting-out of a child on a journey of speech with so small baggage and with so much confidence in the chances of the hedge. He goes free, a simple adventurer. Nor does he make any officious effort to invent anything strange or particularly expressive or descriptive. The child trusts genially to his hearer.

ALICE MEYNELL

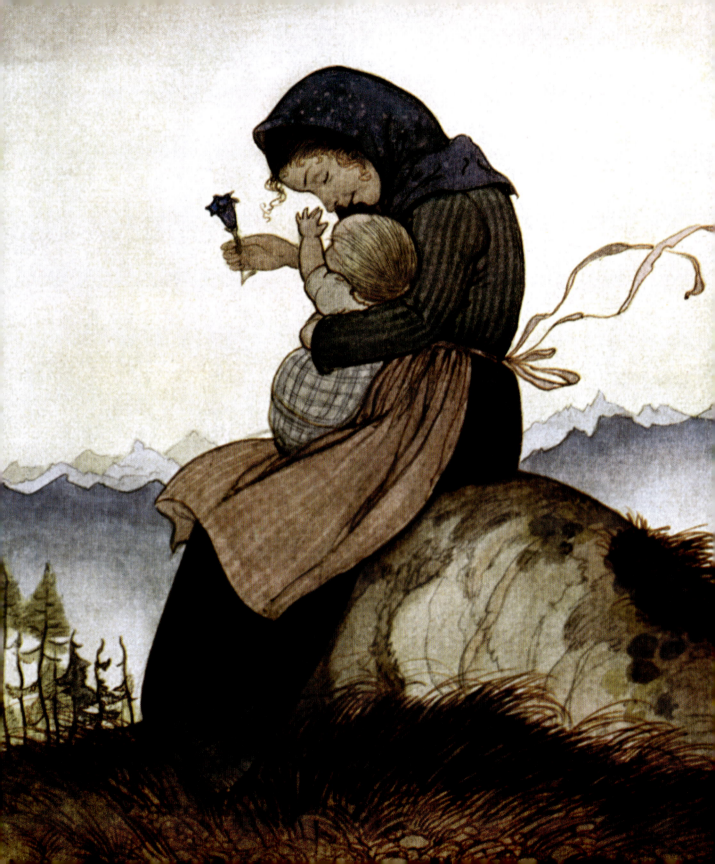

GROWING

Bright soul, new stranded on life's beach,
What wealth of wisdom you might teach
Could we unlock the gates of speech!

Your croonings of that never-land,
Alas! we cannot understand.
We can but kiss your tiny hand.

M.N.D'A.

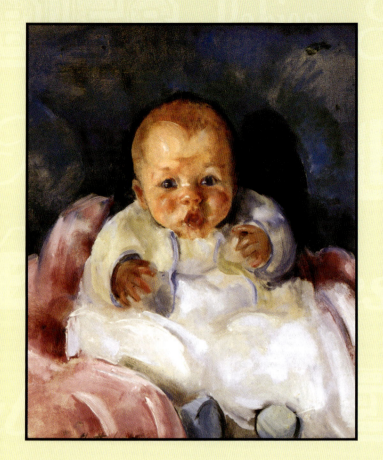

Say papa, baby. Say pa pa pa pa pa pa pa. And baby did his level best to say it for he was very intelligent for eleven months

everyone said and big for his age and the picture of health, a perfect little bunch of

love, and he would certainly turn out to be something great, they said.

—Haja ja ja haja.

JAMES JOYCE

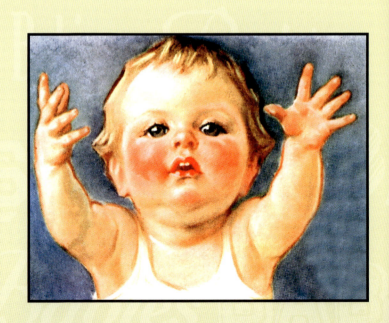

GROWING

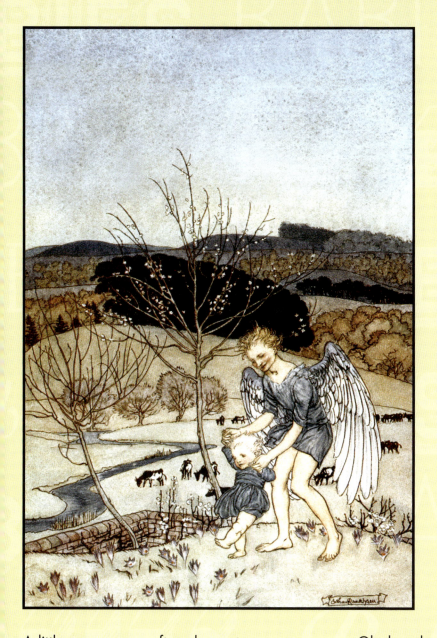

A little way, more soft and sweet
Than fields aflower with May,
A babe's feet, venturing, scarce complete
A little way.

Eyes full of dawning day
Look up for mother's eyes to meet,
Too blithe for song to say.

Glad as the golden spring to greet
Its first live leaflet's play,
Love, laughing, leads the little feet
A little way.

ALGERNON CHARLES SWINBURNE

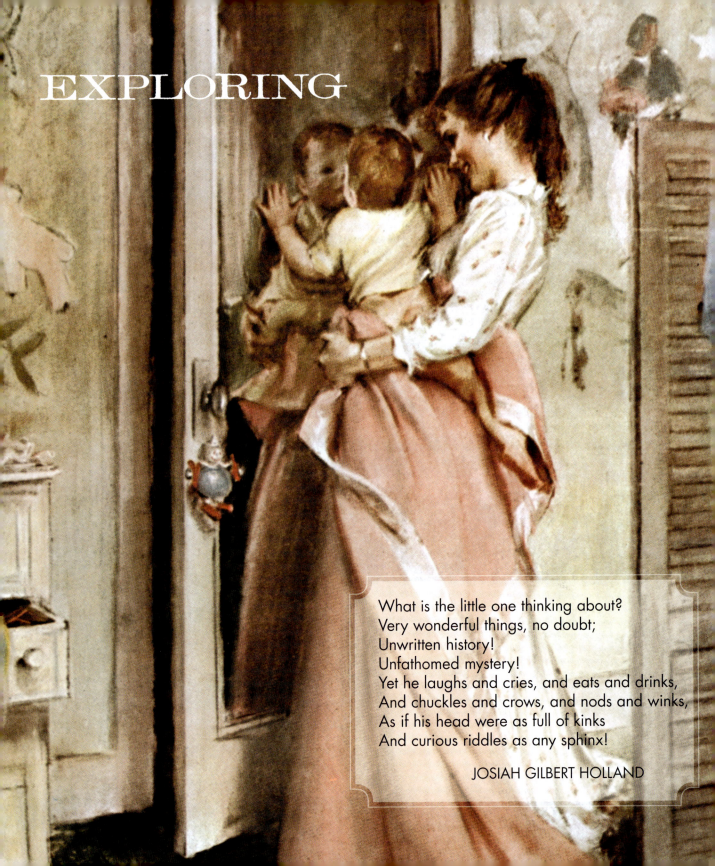

EXPLORING

What is the little one thinking about?
Very wonderful things, no doubt;
Unwritten history!
Unfathomed mystery!
Yet he laughs and cries, and eats and drinks,
And chuckles and crows, and nods and winks,
As if his head were as full of kinks
And curious riddles as any sphinx!

JOSIAH GILBERT HOLLAND

EXPLORING

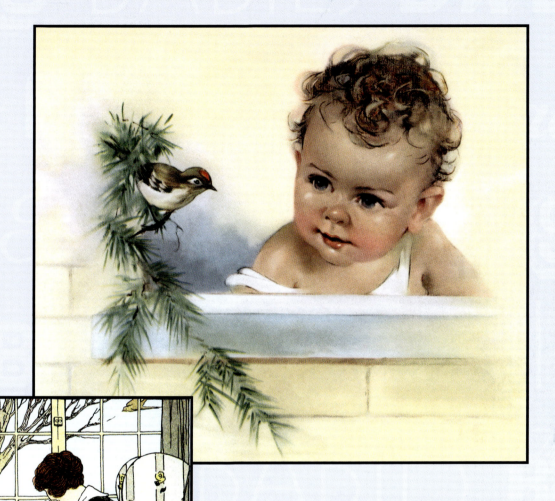

The children's world is full of sweet surprises;
Our common things are precious in their sight:
For them the stars shine, and the morning rises
To show new treasures of untold delight.

SARAH DOUDNEY

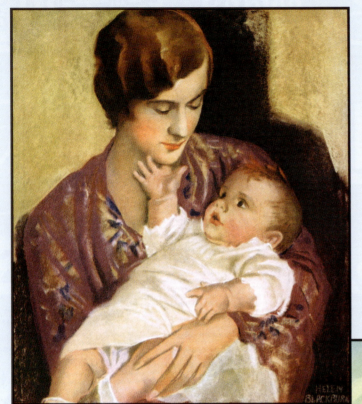

How like an Angel came I down!
  How bright are all things here!
When first among His works I did appear
  O how their glory me did crown!
The world resembled his Eternity,
  In which my soul did walk;
And every thing that I did see
  Did with me talk.

        THOMAS TRAHERNE

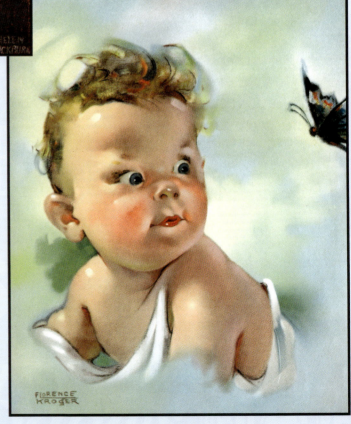

EXPLORING

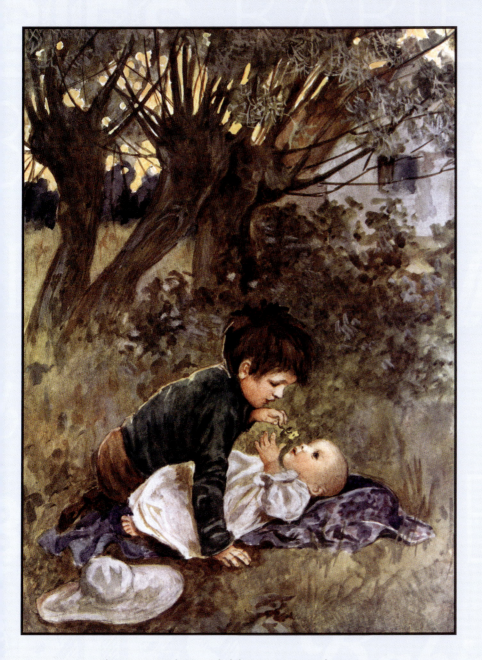

Know you what it is to be a child? … It is to have a spirit yet streaming from the waters of baptism; it is to believe in love, to believe in loveliness, to believe in belief; it is to be so little that the elves can reach to whisper in your ear; it is to turn pumpkins into coaches, and mice into horses, lowness into loftiness, and nothing into everything, for each child has its fairy godmother in its own soul; it is to live in a nutshell and to count yourself the king of infinite space.

FRANCIS THOMPSON

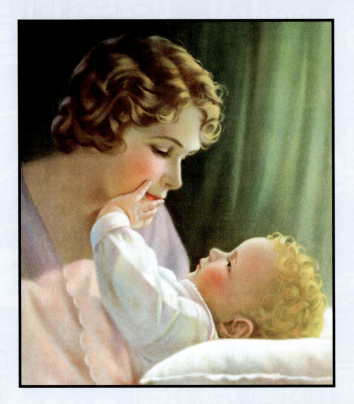

This daylight is for his eyes to open and see. This air is for his lungs to fill themselves with. This earth is for his feet to walk on, and these thoughts are for his brain to go to work on, and these words are for his tongue to start uttering. And these people who have broken into his solitude—they are here to love him and to teach him to love.

THOMAS HOWARD

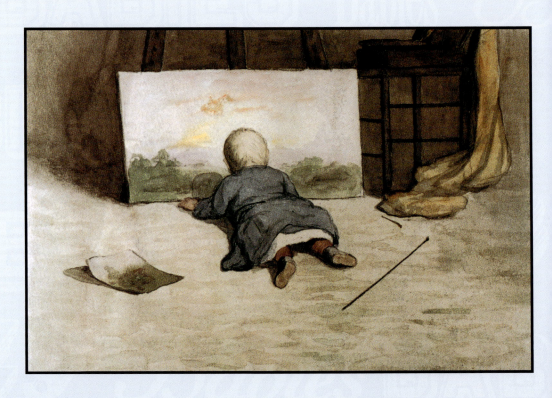

EXPLORING

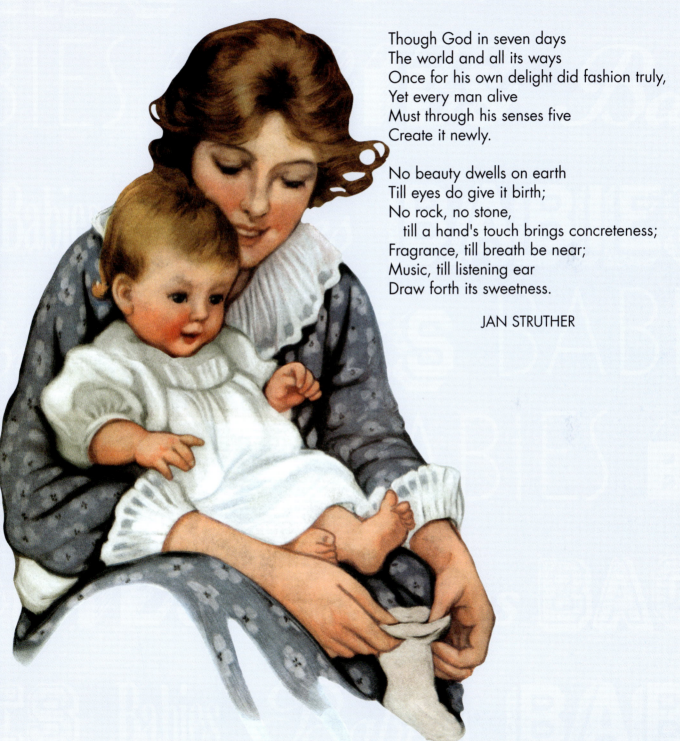

Though God in seven days
The world and all its ways
Once for his own delight did fashion truly,
Yet every man alive
Must through his senses five
Create it newly.

No beauty dwells on earth
Till eyes do give it birth;
No rock, no stone,
 till a hand's touch brings concreteness;
Fragrance, till breath be near;
Music, till listening ear
Draw forth its sweetness.

JAN STRUTHER

BEAUTY

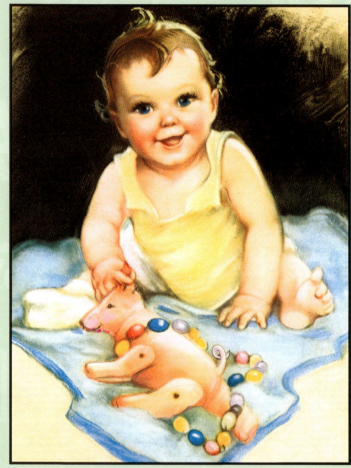

Red, red gold, a kingdom's ransom, child,
To weave thy yellow hair she bade them spin.
At early dawn the gossamer spiders toiled,
And wove the sunrise in.

She took the treasures of the deep blue moon,
She took the clear eyes of the morning star,
The pale-faced lilies of a seven-days moon,
The dust of Phoebus' car.

She painted thee with dewdrops from the flowers,
Stained with their petals, hyacinth and rose,
And violets all wet with April showers,
And snowdrops from the snows.

WILFRID SCAWEN BLUNT

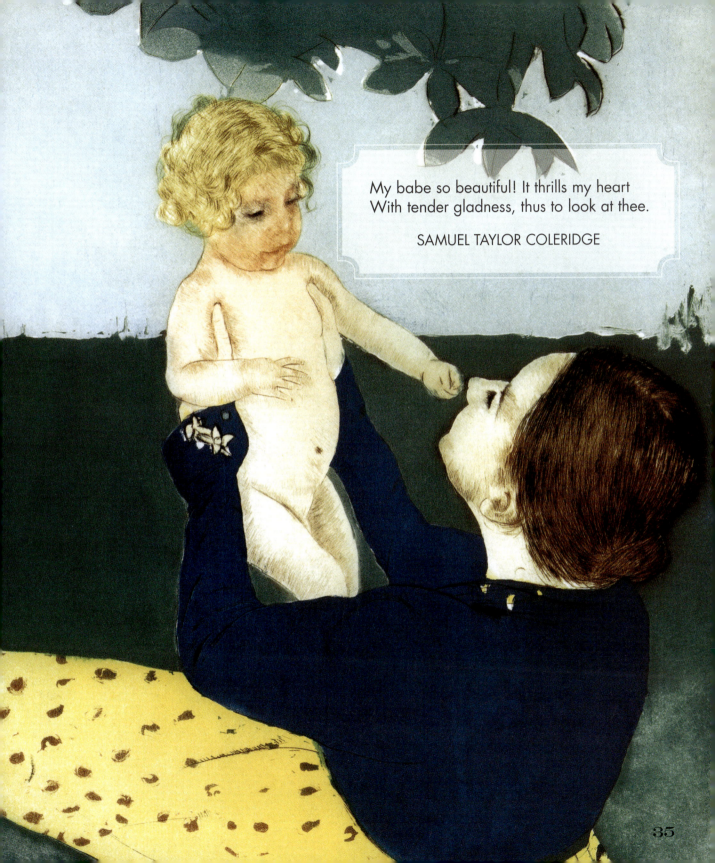

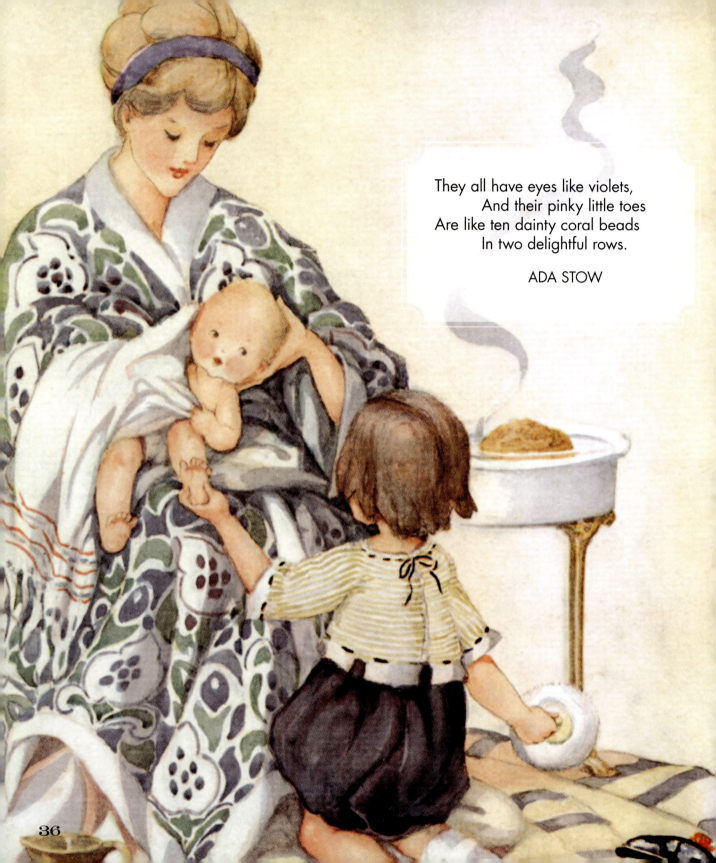

They all have eyes like violets,
And their pinky little toes
Are like ten dainty coral beads
In two delightful rows.

ADA STOW

I have a child; so fair
As golden flowers is she,
My Cleïs, all my care.
I'd not give her away
For Lydia's wide sway
Nor lands men long to see.

    SAPPHO

BEAUTY

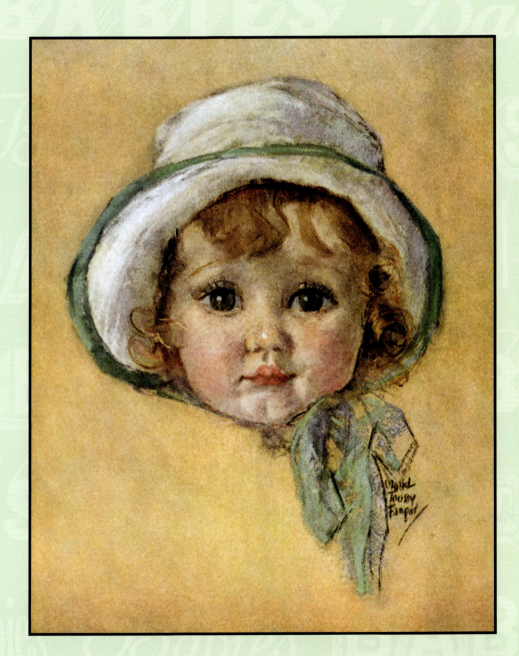

BEAUTY

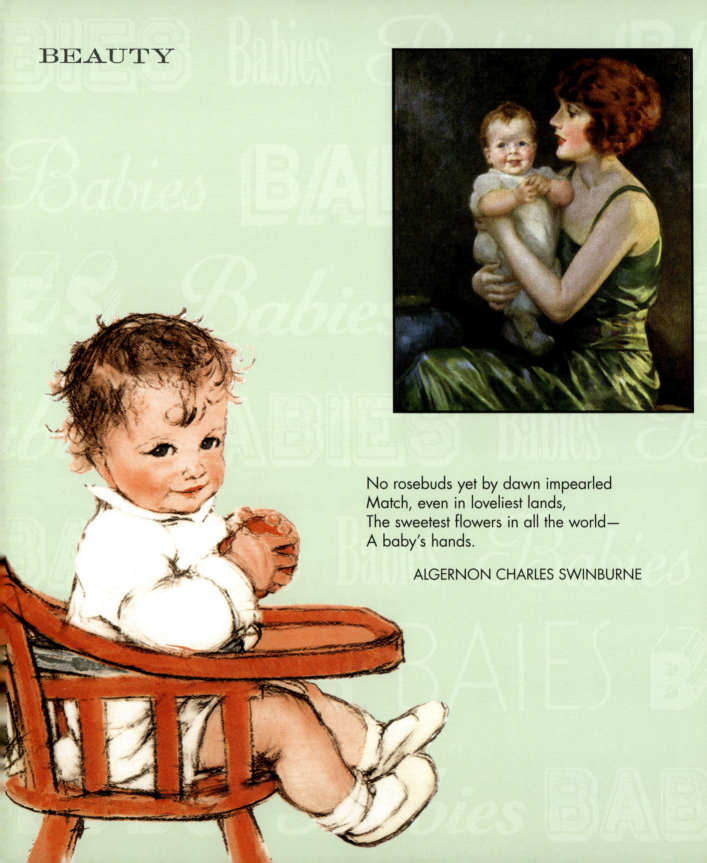

No rosebuds yet by dawn impearled
Match, even in loveliest lands,
The sweetest flowers in all the world—
A baby's hands.

ALGERNON CHARLES SWINBURNE

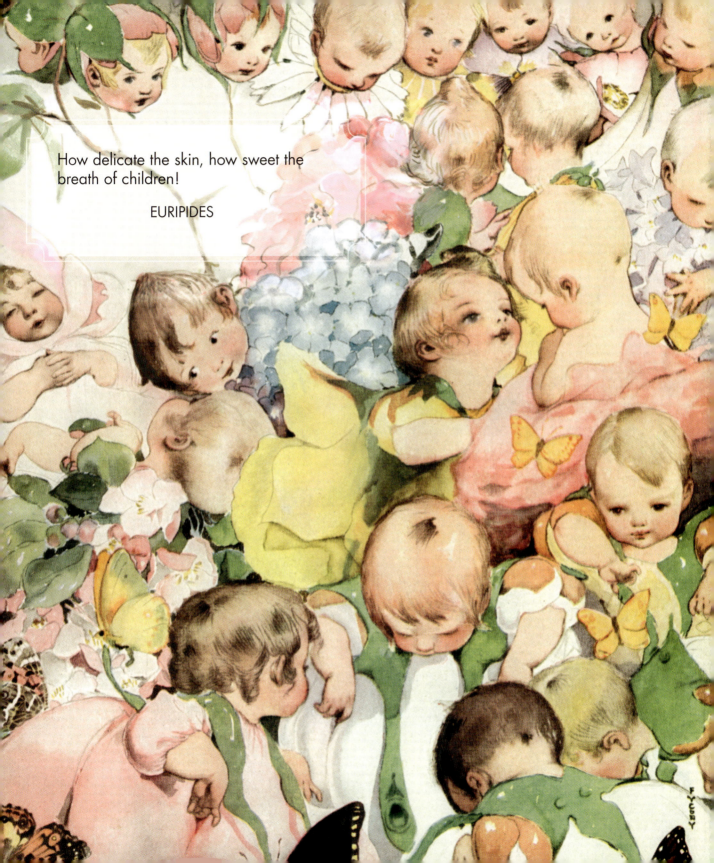

How delicate the skin, how sweet the breath of children!

EURIPIDES

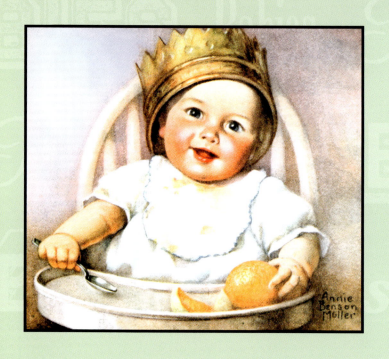

A baby's feet, like sea-shells pink,
  Might tempt, should Heaven see meet,
An angel's lips to kiss, we think,
  A baby's feet.

Like rose-hued sea-flowers toward the heat
  They stretch and spread and wink
Their ten soft buds that part and meet.

ALGERNON CHARLES SWINBURNE

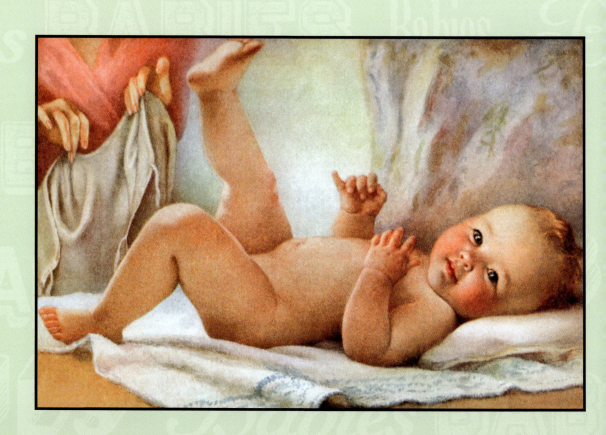

BEAUTY

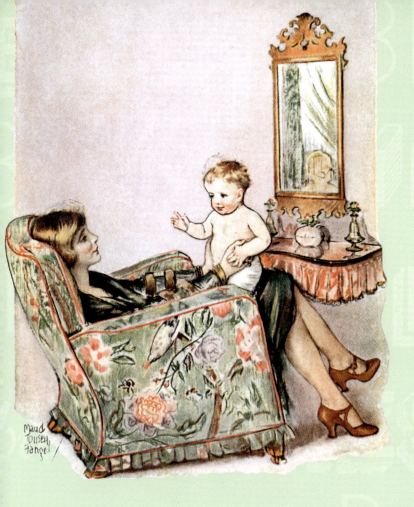

Her shining eyes of sapphire blue
Are like the sky when stars peep through.
Her ears are pretty as some shell
Found in a cave where sea-nymphs dwell.

    MARGARET PAGE

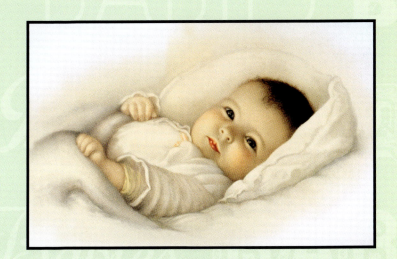

Sweetest little fellow,
Everybody knows:
Don't know what to call him,
But he's mighty like a rose.

Looking for his Mommy
With eyes so shiny blue,
Making you think that heaven
Is coming close to you.

    FRANK L. STANTON

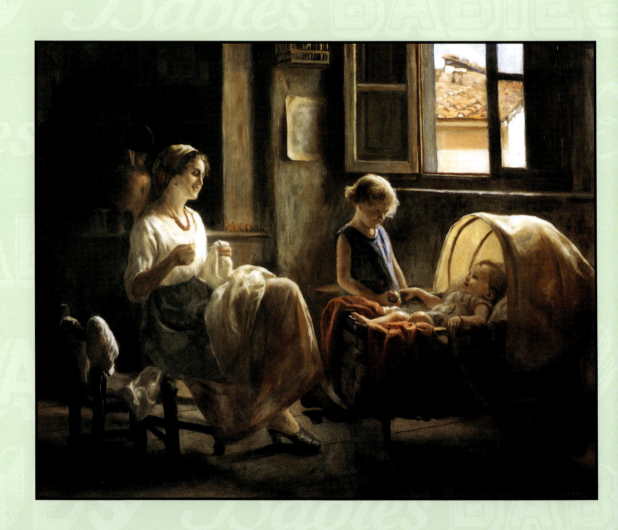

BEAUTY

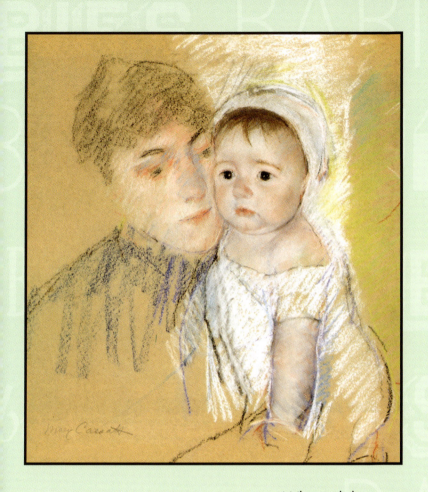

Where did you come from, baby dear?
Out of the everywhere into here.

Where did you get those eyes so blue?
Out of the sky as I came through.

Where did you get that little tear?
I found it waiting when I got here.

What makes your forehead so smooth and high?
A soft hand stroked it as I went by.

What makes your cheek like a warm white rose?
I saw something better than any one knows.

GEORGE MACDONALD

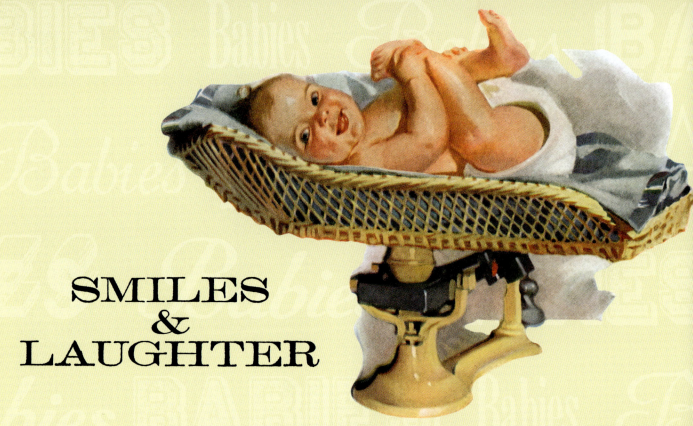

SMILES & LAUGHTER

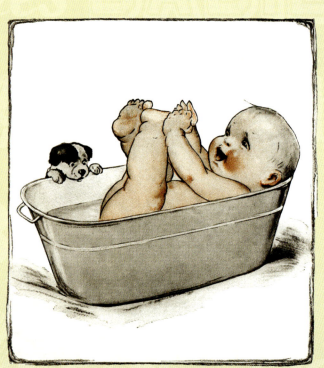

What do they do in Babyland?
Dream and wake, and play,
Laugh and crow,
Shout and grow—
Jolly times have they!

GEORGE COOPER

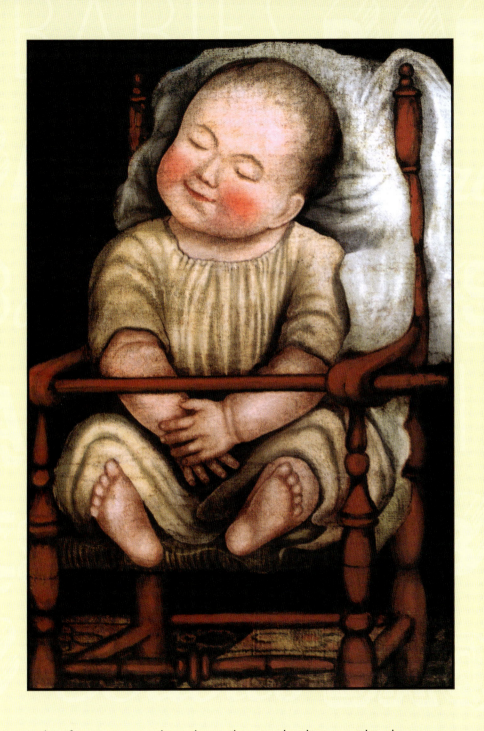

Some, admiring what motives to mirth infants meet with in their silent and solitary smiles, have resolved... that then they converse with angels!

    THOMAS FULLER

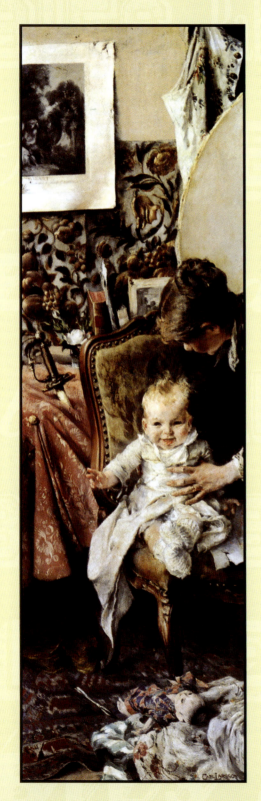

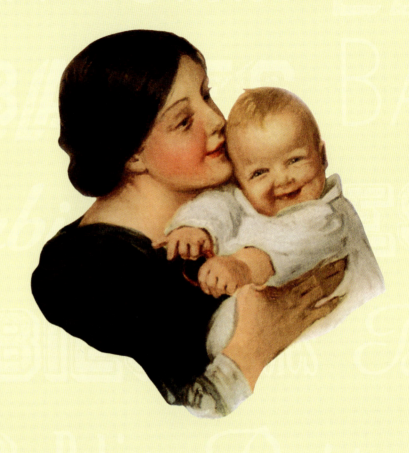

When the first baby laughed for the first time, the laugh broke into a thousand pieces and they all went skipping about, and that was the beginning of fairies.

JAMES BARRIE

SMILES & LAUGHTER

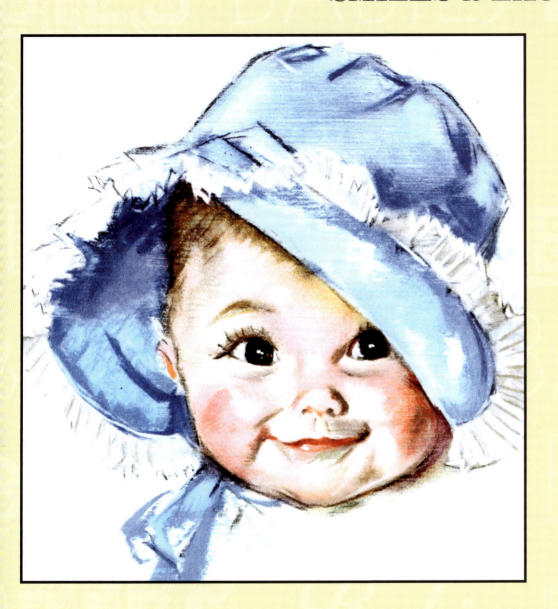

My baby cries—and All the world is wrong.
My baby laughs—The world is full of song.

HINDUSTANI SAYING

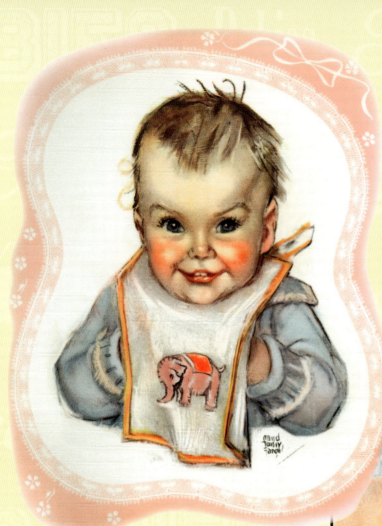

Children in the wind– hair floating, tossing, a miniature of the agitated trees below which they played. The elder whirling for joy the one in petticoats, a fat baby, eddying half-willingly, half by the force of the gust, driven backward, struggling forward both drunk with the pleasure, both shouting their hymn of joy.

SAMUEL TAYLOR COLERIDGE

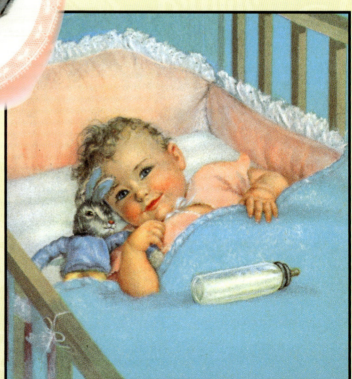

SMILES & LAUGHTER

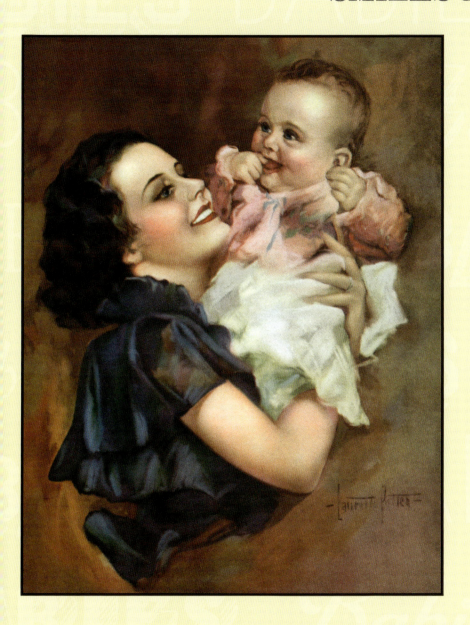

She was a very happy child, and once she learned to smile, she never stopped; at first she would smile at anything, at parking meters and dogs and strangers, but as she grew older she began to favour me, and nothing gave me more delight than her evident preference.

MARGARET DRABBLE

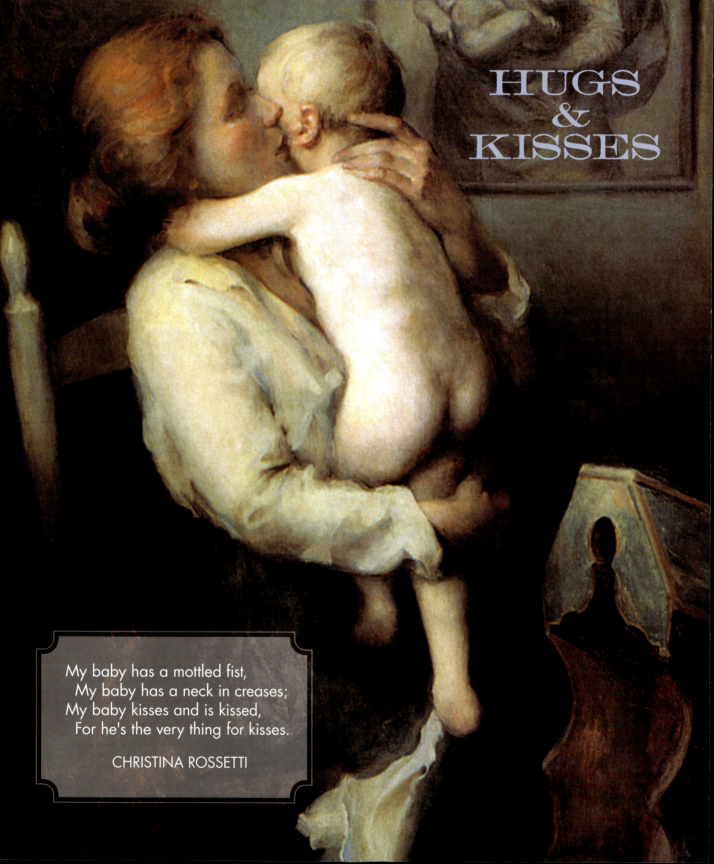

HUGS & KISSES

My baby has a mottled fist,
　My baby has a neck in creases;
My baby kisses and is kissed,
　For he's the very thing for kisses.

CHRISTINA ROSSETTI

HUGS & KISSES

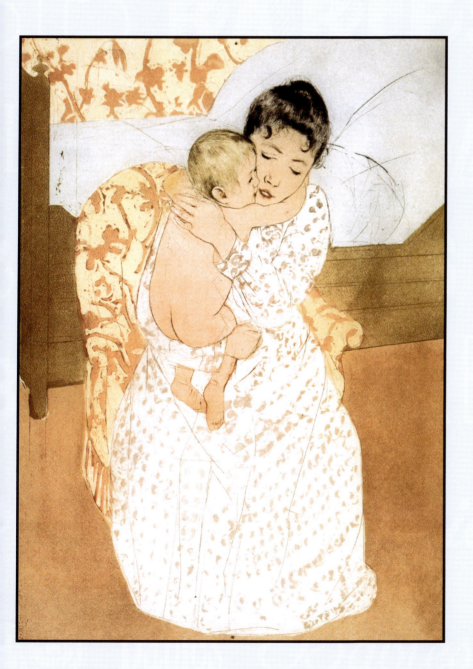

Sweet babe, in thy face,
Soft desires I can trace,
Secret joys and secret smiles,
Little pretty infant wiles.

    WILLIAM BLAKE

"Cuddle and love me, cuddle and love me,"
Crows the mouth of coral pink:
Oh, the bald head, and, oh, the sweet lips,
And, oh, the sleepy eyes that wink!

    CHRISTINA ROSSETTI

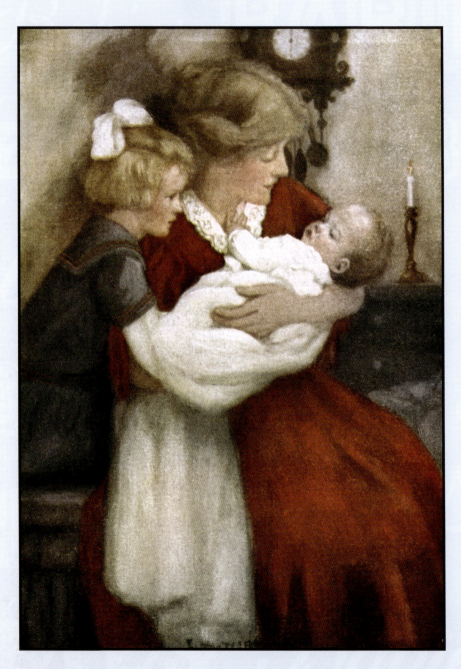

HUGS & KISSES

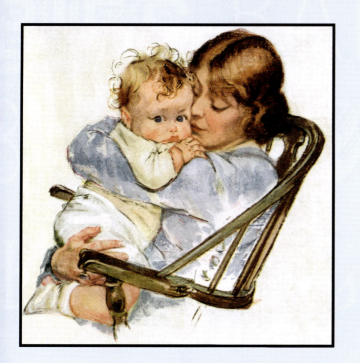

A little child born yesterday,
A thing on mother's milk and kisses fed.

HOMER

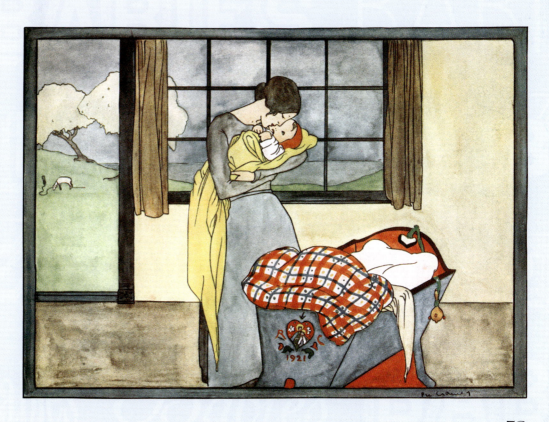

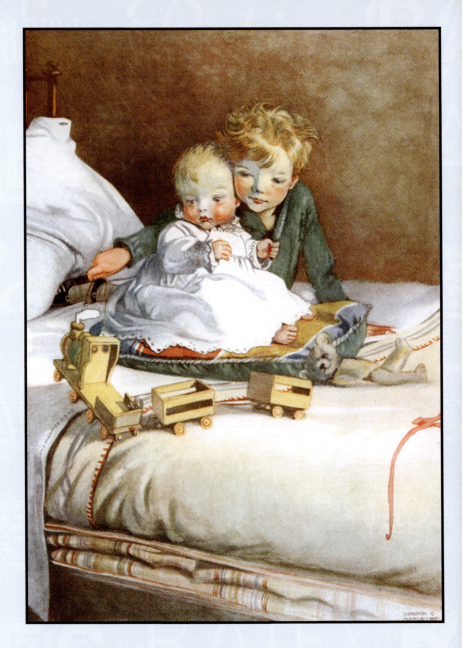

I love you well, my little brother,
And you are fond of me;
Let us be kind to one another,
As brothers ought to be.

You shall learn to play with me,
And learn to use my toys;
And then I think that we shall be
Two happy little boys.

    UNKNOWN

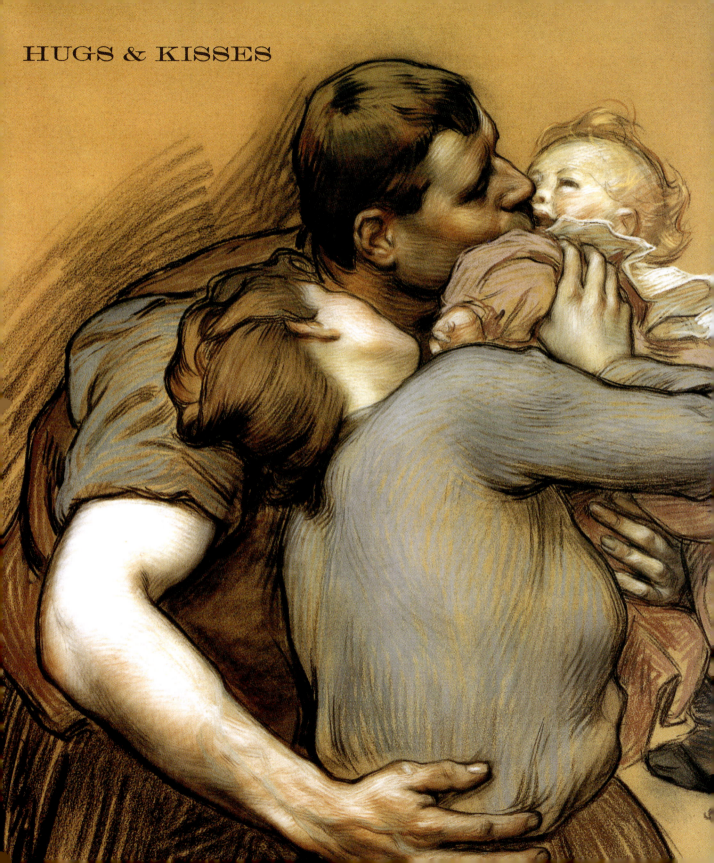

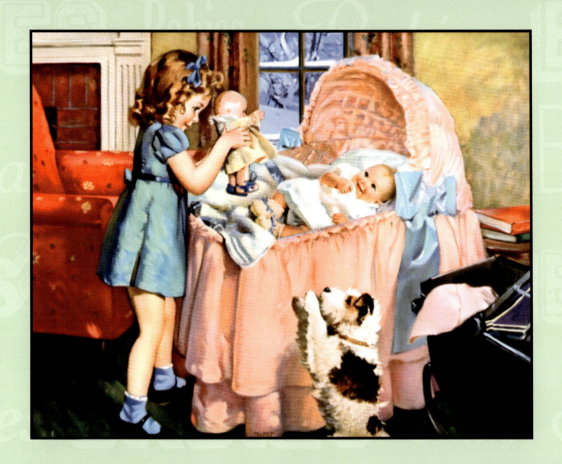

All The
LOVEABLE
Rest

A dreary place would this earth be
Were there no little people in it;
The song of life would lose its mirth,
Were there no children to begin it.

No forms, like buds, to grow,
And make the admiring heart surrender;
No little hands on breast and brow,
To keep the thrilling love-chords tender.

The sterner souls would grow more stern,
Unfeeling nature more inhuman,
And man to stoic coldness turn,
And woman would be less than woman.

Life's song, indeed, would lose its charm
Were there no babies to begin it;
A doleful place this world would be,
Were there no little people in it.

JOHN GREENLEAF WHITTIER

LOVEABLE

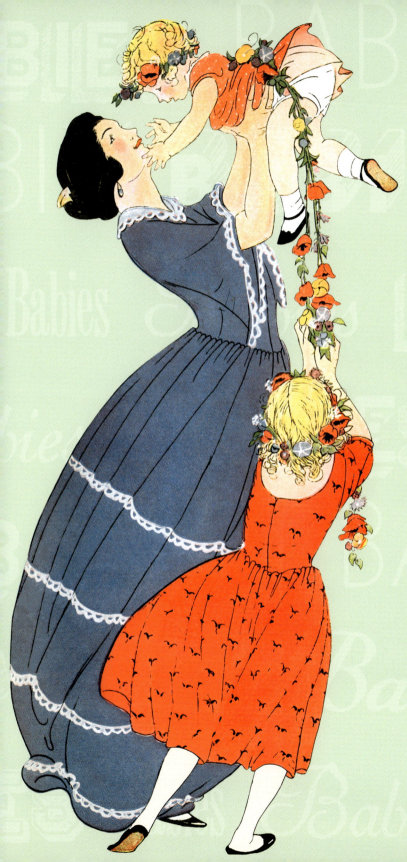

"I have no name:
I am but two days old."
What shall I call thee?
"I happy am,
Joy is my name."
Sweet joy befall thee!

Pretty joy!
Sweet joy but two days old,
Sweet joy I call thee;
Thou dost smile,
I sing the while;
Sweet joy befall thee!

   WILLIAM BLAKE

The world has no such flowers in any land,
And no such pearl in any gulf the sea,
As any babe on any mother's knee.

PELAGIUS

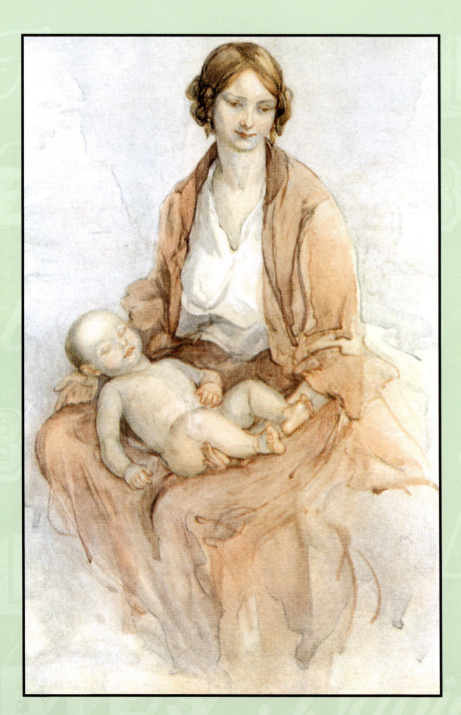

LOVEABLE

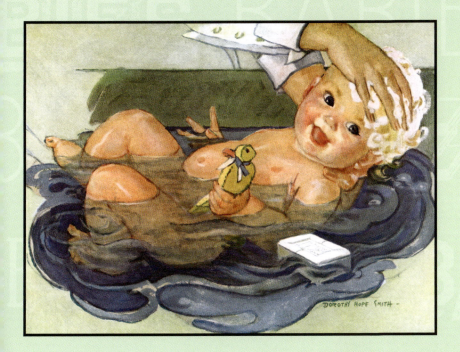

Baby wakes up in the morning light;
Pick her up and hold her tight.
Put little baby in the tub—
Scrubbity, scrubbity, scrub-scrub!
Squeeze the sponge and use the soap—
Baby's cool and clean (we hope!)
Dress her up in pretty clothes,
Then outside to play she goes.
Carry her, swing her, sing her a song—
We care for baby all day long!

ERNEST NISTER

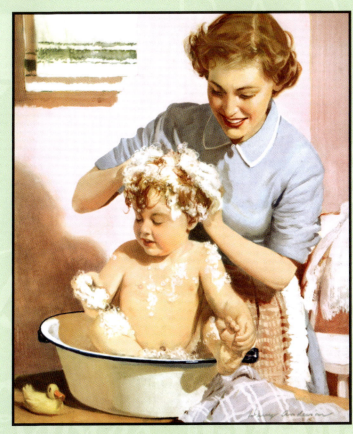

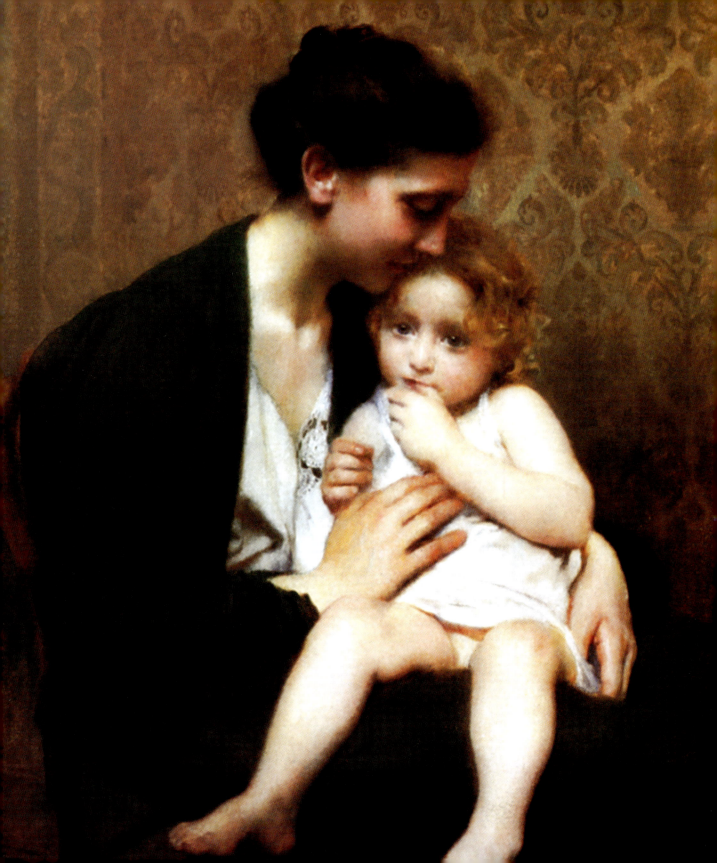

LOVEABLE

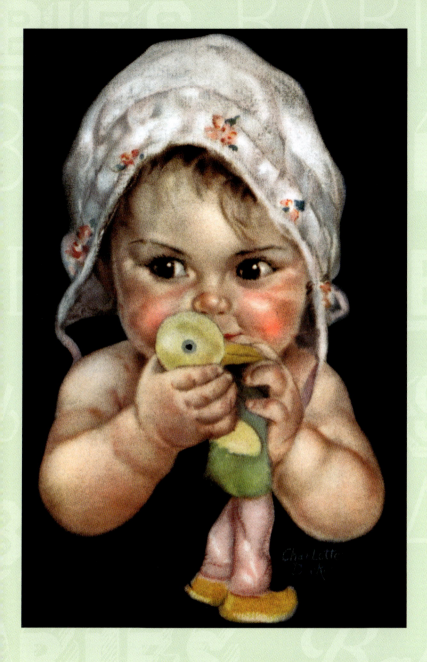

We can all be more or less warm— with fur, with skating, with tea, with fire, and with sleep-in the winter. But the child is fresh in the wind, and wakes cool from his dreams, dewy when there is hoar-frost everywhere else; he is "more lovely and more temperate" than the summer day and than the winter day alike. He overcomes both heat and cold by another climate, which is the climate of life.

    ALICE MEYNELL

Bright soul, new stranded on life's beach,
What wealth of wisdom you might teach
Could we unlock the gates of speech!

Your croonings of that never-land,
Alas! we cannot understand.
We can but kiss your tiny hand.

      M.N.D'A.

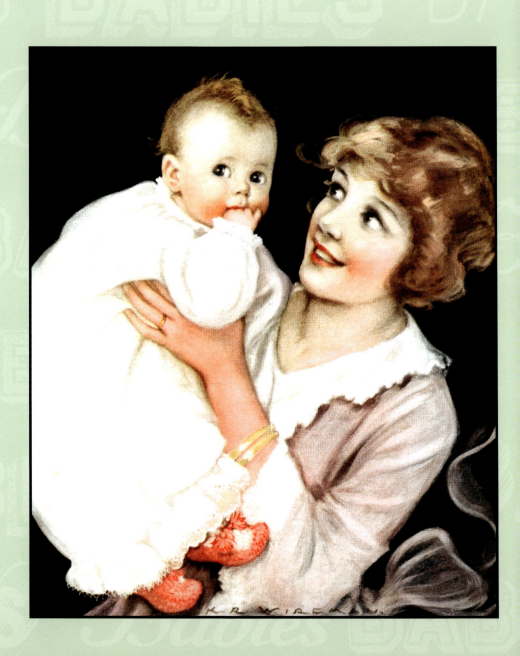

LOVEABLE

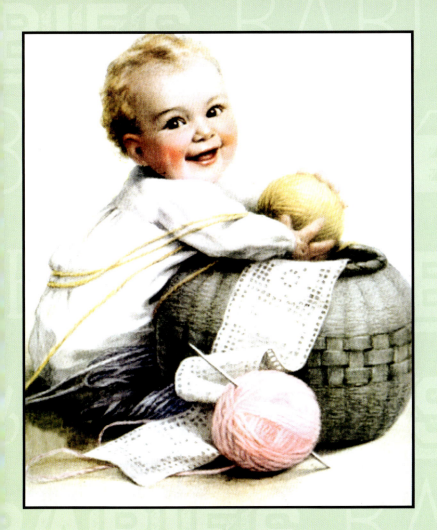

Oh! stupid grown-up people who think yourselves so wise,
If you only saw what I see—saw with a baby's eyes!

You think the baby's laughing at the sunshine on the floor,
But the baby sees the Little Folk dancing by the score.

(A baby's half a fairy and knows all fairy tricks,
But he has quite forgotten by the time he's half-past six.)

FRANCES HODGSON BURNETT

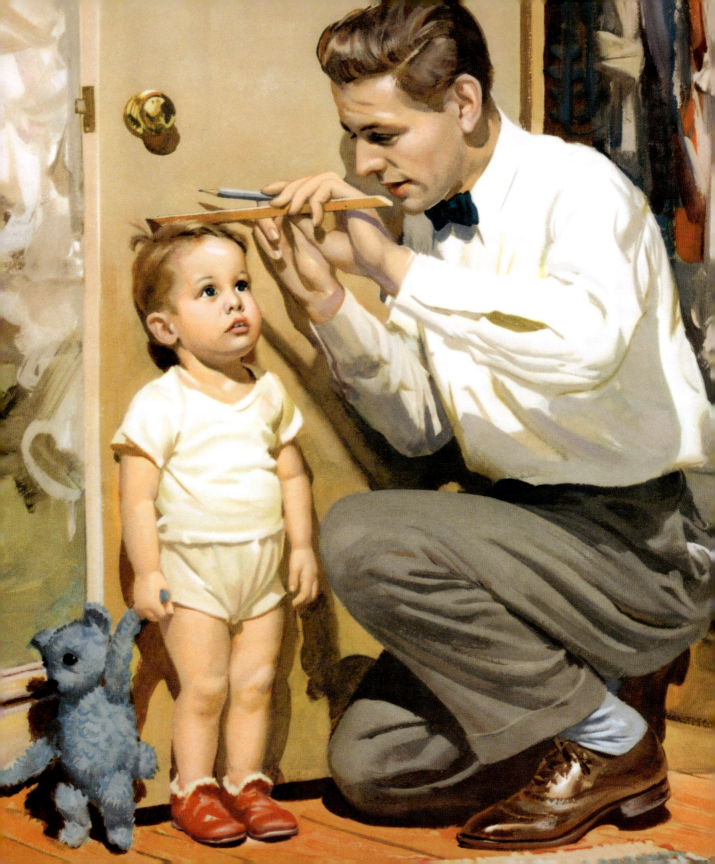

LOVEABLE

I love these little people, and it is not a slight thing when they, fresh from God, love us.

CHARLES DICKENS

PICTURE CREDITS

Cover	E.N. Donaldson. Magazine cover, 1921.
Endpapers	Charles Robinson. Magazine illustration, 1914.
Half Title	Maude Tousey Fangel. Magazine cover, 1933.
Frontispiece	Unknown. Advertising illustration, 1915.
Title Page	Maude Tousey Fangel. Magazine illustration, 1934.
Copyright	Willy Pogany. Magazine illustration, n.d.
2	Guy Hoff. Magazine illustration, n.d.
3	Harrison Fisher. Magazine cover, 1911.
4	(upper) William Adolphe Bouguereau. "Le Reveil," 1865. (lower) Unknown. Advertising illustration, 1939.
5	Ada W. Shulz. "Motherhood," c. 1925.
6	(upper) Frederick William Elwell. "The First Born", 1913. (lower) The Reeses. Magazine advertisement, 1930.
7	John Gannam. Advertising illustration, 1949.
8	(upper) S.D. Runyan. From *Baby's History,* 1908. (lower) Ethel P.B. Leach. "Mother and Child," 1915.
9	John Newton Howitt. Advertising illustration, n.d.
10	S.D. Runyan. From *Baby's History,* 1908.
11	(upper) Thomas Benjamin Kennington. "Maternity," 1897. (lower) Louis-Emile Adan. "La Maternité," 1898.
12	John Gannam. Advertising illustration, n.d.
13	F.Y. Cory. Magazine cover, n.d.
14	(upper) Maud Tousey Fangel. Magazine illustration, 1923. (lower) Andrew Loomis. Magazine illustration, 1925.
15	Anonymous. Magazine illustration, 1922.
16	Allene J. Love. "Darling Asleep," 1936.
17	(upper) Friedrich von Amerling. "Portrait of Princess Marie Franziska von Liechtenstein," 1836. (lower) Maude Tousey Fangel. Magazine illustration, n.d.
18	Unknown. Advertising illustration, 1943.
19	Clara M. Burd. From *Baby's Record,* c. 1921.
20	(upper) Charlotte Becker and Ellen Segner. From *Peter's Family,* 1942. (lower) Unknown. Advertising illustration, n.d.
21	Rose O'Neill. Magazine cover, 1910.
22	Alphaeus-Philemon Cole. "The First Look," n.d.
23	Unknown. Advertising illustration, 1931.
24	Else Wenz-Viëtor. From *Hinter den Sieben Bergen,* 1931.
25	George T. Tobin. Magazine cover, 1909.
26	(upper) Martha Walter. "Baby in White Gown," n.d. (lower) Unknown. Advertising illustration, n.d.
27	Arthur Rackham. From *The Springtide of Life,* 1918.
28	John Gannam. Advertising illustration, 1953.
29	(upper) Florence Kroger. Advertising illustration, 1944. (lower) Blanche Fisher Wright. From *A Baby's Journal,* 1916.
30	(upper) Helen Blackburn. Magazine illustration, n.d. (lower) Florence Kroger. Calendar illustration, n.d.

PICTURE CREDITS

31	Unknown. From *Blackie's Children's Annual 9th Year*, c. 1910.
32	(upper) Unknown. Calendar illustration, c. 1930. (lower) R.B. Gruelle. Untitled watercolor, n.d.
33	Katharine R. Wireman. Magazine cover, 1920.
34	Eleanor Campbell. Illustration, n.d.
35	Mary Cassatt. "Under the Horse-Chestnut Tree," c. 1895.
36	Anne Anderson. Book illustration, n.d.
37	Maud Tousey Fangel. Magazine cover, 1934.
38	(upper) Unknown. Advertising illustration 1924. (lower) Unknown. Advertising illustration, n.d.
39	F.Y. Cory. Magazine cover, 1909.
40	(upper) Annie Benson Müller. Advertising illustration, 1934. (lower) Annie Benson Müller. Magazine illustration, 1934.
41	(upper) Maud Tousey Fangel. Advertising illustration, 1927. (lower) Unknown. "Heaven's Gift," 1932.
42	Giuseppe Magni. "Admiring the Baby," n.d.
43	Mary Cassatt. "Baby Bill in His cap and Shift, Held by His Nurse," c. 1890.
44	(upper) Unknown. Advertising illustration, 1930. (lower) Unknown. Magazine illustration, n.d.
45	Unknown folk artist. "Baby in Red Chair," c. 1800.
46	(right) Unknown. Advertising illustration, 1919. (left) Carl Larsson. "Lille Suzanne," 1885.
47	Maud Tousey Fangel. Illustration, n.d.
48	(upper) Maud Tousey Fangel. From *Babies*, 1933. (lower) Unknown. "A Little Bit of Heaven," n.d.
49	Laurent Potter. Calendar illustration, n.d.
50	Marion Boyd Allen. "Motherhood," 1920.
51	Mary Cassatt. "Nude Child," 1890.
52	Eugenie Wireman. From *Yourself and Your House Wonderful*, 1913.
53	(upper) Unknown. Advertising illustration, 1923. (lower) Rie Cramer. From *Little Dutchy*, 1925.
54	Honor C. Appleton. From *The Bower Book*, 1922.
55	Victor Prouvé. Untitled drawing, c. 1898.
56	F. Sands Brunner. Calendar illustration, 1949.
57	Maginel Wright Enright. Magazine illustration, 1923.
58	Bess Norriss. "An Autumn Portrait," n.d.
59	(upper) Dorothy Hope Smith. Advertising illustration, 1932. (lower) Harry Anderson. Calendar illustration, n.d.
60	Paul LeRoy. "Maternity, " 1899.
61	Charlotte Becker. "The Flirt," n.d.
62	Katherine R. Wireman. Magazine cover, 1922.
63	Annie Benson Müller. Magazine cover, 1922.
64	Harry Anderson. Calendar illustration, n.d.
65	S.D. Runyon. Illustration, 1908.
68	Marie Madeleine Franc-Nohain. From *La Journal de Bébé*, 1914.
Back Cover	Friedrich von Amerling. "Portrait of Princess Karoline von Liechtenstein," 1837.

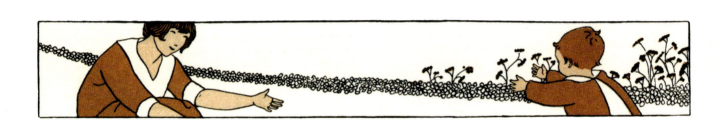